Alabi Fidelix Aigbona

The Hungry Hunter

AF889932

Alabi Fidelix Aigbona

The Hungry Hunter

Discover you and your talent

Blessed Hope Publishing

Imprint

Any brand names and product names mentioned in this book are subject to trademark, brand or patent protection and are trademarks or registered trademarks of their respective holders. The use of brand names, product names, common names, trade names, product descriptions etc. even without a particular marking in this work is in no way to be construed to mean that such names may be regarded as unrestricted in respect of trademark and brand protection legislation and could thus be used by anyone.

Cover image: www.ingimage.com

Publisher:
Blessed Hope Publishing
is a trademark of
International Book Market Service Ltd., member of OmniScriptum Publishing Group
17 Meldrum Street, Beau Bassin 71504, Mauritius
Printed at: see last page
ISBN: 978-613-7-89929-8

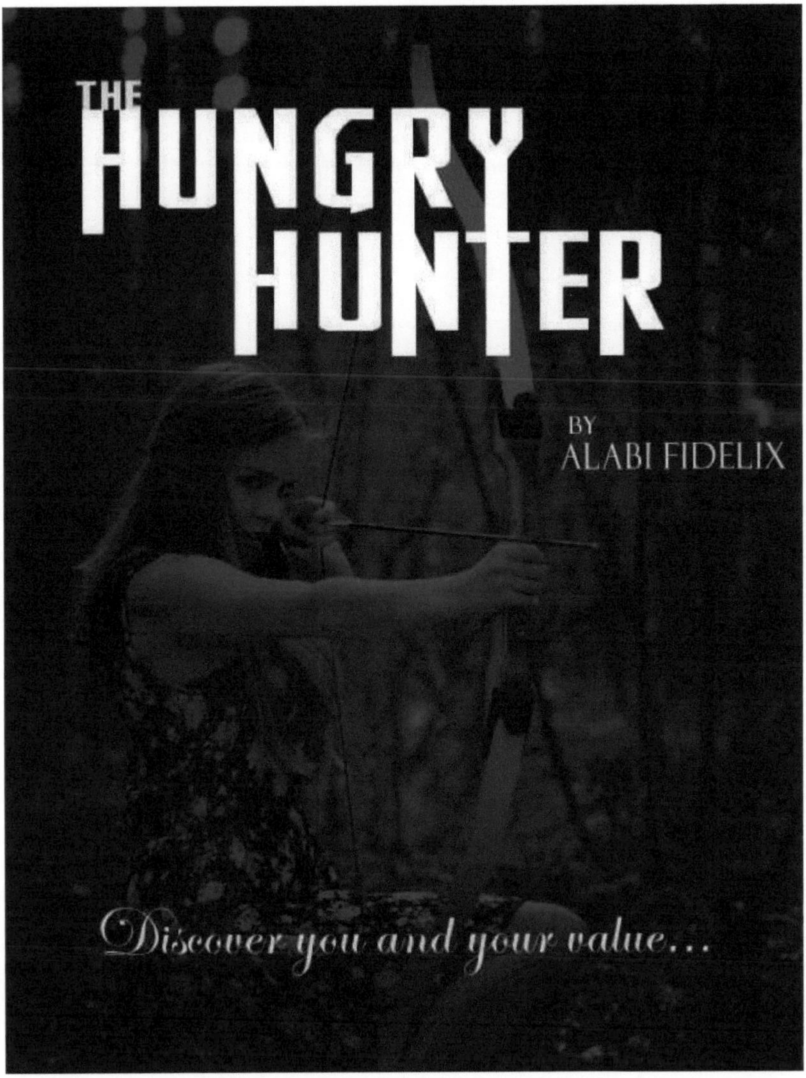
THE
HUNGRY
HUNTER
BY
ALABI FIDELIX
Discover you and your value...

Acknowledgement

I want to thank God Almighty for giving me the grace to author this book, I say may His name alone be praised. I want to cease this opportunity to thank everyone who had contributed to making this book a reality, I say God bless you. I want to appreciate my daddy Pastor J.K. Omonije who took time to proof read my book, indeed you are a father. I also want to appreciate the Senior Pastor of my church Pastor Ugoh Andrew and his wife with our District Youth Coordinator in person of Pastor Chris Olodefadehan and his wife. I won't fail to acknowledge a friend my best friend, Princess Oyegbile Oluwaseun. Most importantly, I appreciate the person God use to bring this book into reality. It's no other person than Pst Engr Femi Oduwole with his wife, God bless you all.

TABLE OF CONTENTS

Introduction

In life there is always cause and effect, what you do today has the tendency to influence what happens tomorrow. It is so disheartening to see a lot of people selling out their valuable values that will have made their life worthwhile tomorrow. This action has resulted to poverty that has knocked so many people down, and set homes and nations to go begging in our today's world.

Ignorance and family background have driven many people into disvaluing their values. The set of values and principles an individual gets acquainted with while growing up have a subtle way of influencing the quality of his/her decision through life. Of course, you are not left out of this. In the long run, these decisions also have a way of determining your future. Several times have I made people understand that when diagnosis to a particular problem is wrong, prescription will automatically be wrong; one day in a chemistry class I approached my teacher and told him that the chemical equation we are to balance is not correct. I have tried every method I knew to balance the equation without arriving at the answer so I said to the teacher, 'sir the equation is wrong'. The teacher said to me 'Fidelix' go and work it out again. I sat for some time going through the work and I still cannot get to the answer so I stood up to meet him again. And he said Fidelix you are lazy there is no problem with the equation. While I stood arguing with my teacher, he called one of my classmates to come forward and show his work to me. I moved closer to see it hoping to find him in the same predicament I was in. I was disappointed. He had arrived at the answer my teacher said we would arrive at. To hide my face I retorted, "sir, this balancing of equation is too difficult". And my teacher looked at me and said "it is not the equation that is difficult but your equation which is weak". I turned with embarrassment and feel very stupid. The question was not wrong but it was my strength in balancing equations that was weak. It follows that **when your perception towards your own value is wrong, developing it to better your life will also be wrong**.

Esau's and Jacob's prodigy was a case study in this book. Your understanding in reading this book will define how wonderful and glorious your future will look like. It is easy to wave hunger off when the present alone is considered however with the future in view, say the next five, ten or twenty years; what appears trivial now will be seen in a different light. Do you know what **the Hungry Hunter** is all about? Follow me as I explore the scripture to making the folded unfold.

Foreword

This book, The Hungry Hunter is both revealing and challenging for everyone who desires to leave a foot print on the sand of time.
The sharp contrast between Esau's and Jacob's lifestyle is a wakeup call to everyone.
It is possible to be a hardworking person and still fail woefully. Someone else can choose to be a smart, good working person and succeed greatly.
Esau had lots of potentials yet he lacked discipline to turn around his potentials into outstanding achievement and fulfilment of destiny. He lacked patience and endurance to turn his life around. He had all it takes to successfully hunt a game but lack a little more patience, discipline and endurance to roast his game. What a tragedy.

On the other hand, Jacob, who looked to be lazy on the outside had the wisdom of an investor, the energy of a youth, the skill of a craft man, the knowledge of the educated, homesick lessness of the sailor, the focus of the pilot, and of course the devotion of the preacher and beat the tape of success.

As a matter of fact, everyone must learn how to process his/her gifts and talents, know how to package, brand and rebrand every endowment of yours if you must stand out, enhance your value and become sought for in life.
This takes all round discipline: discipline of clear thinking, discipline of daily goal setting, of daily time management, periodic saving and investing, of continuous learning and, of course, discipline of persistence.

The third world nations, most especially, a nation as ours (Nigeria) need to wake up. Let's go extra mile to turn all our natural resources around to enhance our wealth and make the country worth living for all.
This book is a must read for everyone including decision makers of third-world nations. It is an eye opener for success and breakthrough.

Evang Omonije J. K

Chapter 1

ESAU AND JACOB

Jacob and Esau were brothers, twin brothers, the sons of Isaac and Rebekah and grandsons of Abraham, the great patriarch of the Jewish. Normally twins are a whole lot alike, they dress alike, they act alike, they even think alike.

Esau and Jacob are different and they differ in their appearance, they differ in pursuit, they differ in thinking and they differ in character. Let quickly read the bible (Gen. 25:27-34) AMP.

27 When the boys grew up, Esau was a cunning and skilled hunter, a man of outdoor(field); but Jacob was a plane and quit man dwelling in tent.

28 And Isaac loved (and was partial to...) Esau because he ate of Esau's game; but Rebekah loved Jacob.

29 Jacob was boiling pottage (lentil stew) one day, when Esau came from the field and was faint (with hunger).

30 And Esau said to Jacob, I beg of you, let me have some of that lentil stew to eat, for I am faint and famished that was why his name was called Edom (Red).

31 Jacob answered, then sell me today your birthright (the right of a firstborn).

32 Esau said, see here, I am at the point of death; what good can this birthright do me?

33Jacob said, swear to me today (that you are selling it to me); and he swore to (Jacob) and sold his birthright.

34And Jacob gave Esau bread and stew of lentils and he ate and drank and rose up and went his way thus Esau scorned his birthright as beneath his notice.

In the verses, we see two things

- **Birthright And**
- **The Barter**

THE BIRTHRIGHT: like the name implies, was the right of the first-born son in the family to receive his father's inheritance upon his father's death. But there was more to the BIRTHRIGHT than just financial gain. With the birthright came the blessing. This typically went to the firstborn as well. The point in this birthright is something to be valued and treasured. Even thou Jacob and Esau were twins, Esau had "the BIRTHRIGHT" because he was born first.

THE BARTER: the barter is one you don't hear very often these days but there was a time when great deals of business transaction were carried out by "bartering". To **barter** simply means to "trade", to exchange goods or services for goods or services. On that day Esau and Jacob engage in a little bartering.

Many sermons have been preached about the story of Esau and Jacob, most of the story heard, was how Jacob cheated on his brother for the birthright or whenever the chapter of this story was read, everybody's mind will go to predestination.

One day Esau came in from hunting trip, he was tired and he his starving. In studying the lives of Esau and Jacob my attention was caught on verse 30 of the book Genesis chapter 25.

"And Esau said to Jacob, I beg of you, let me have some of that red lentil stew to eat, for I am faint and famished. That was why his name was called Edom (red)".

If any should be hungry, I thought it should be Jacob because he stayed in the tent and did not go out to hunt for food. The one who works harder in the field has no food to eat but the one who stays in the tent is cooking a stew. Esau is a skillful man who cannot do without killing a prey on any venture he went for.

SKILLS OF A HUNTER

As a hunter, you must have the following skills:

- ★ **Ability to tiptoe:** A good hunter must know how to work with his toe so as to avoid giving signal to prey of his approach. Hunters are silent in movement and quick on the feet.
- ★ **Ability to locate prey: Hunters** are predictors. A good hunter studies the movement of his prey. He should be able to interpret track of an animal even if it is made week past. Should be able to know where to find what he is looking for.
- ★ **Ability to pursue: A** hunter must be a good runner. He or she must have the physical inbuilt strength and stamina that enables him to run after what he's looking for. A Hunter know how to stalk his prey until he's able to strike.
- ★ **Ability to kill: P**ursuit of the animal is expected to end in becoming a prey for the hunter.

- ★ **Take home:** After all the chasing and killing of the prey, the hunter must know how to bring it home.
- ★ **Above all he must be able to roast his game to make it edible.**

Esau kind of people happened to be the hard-working people of the world today but never seems to have enough to feed themselves and their family let alone saving. They work hard in field such as hospital, school, music, industries like mining, agricultural and companies of various kinds but never have enough to liberate themselves from economic dependency. Why? This set of people thinks the way to a better life is simply to work hard and wear themselves off. As a result of that point of view, they focus all their productive priorities on putting on extra hour and effort without ever stopping to think about how to redesign and organize their working structure with strategies. They take so much delight or pride in how much God has blessed them with resources yet have very little to show for their pride. I happened to be among this set of people before. I worked from Monday to Saturday 6:30am to 8:00pm sometimes 9:00pm everyday but I have little to show for it until I discovered that **"it is not all about struggling but it is all about strategies"**. Have you noticed that some of the richest country or nations today are strangely not endowed with natural resources while some of the poorest nations in the world today, are also strangely the most richly endowed in natural resources? The land mass of their country or nation have vast deposits of gold, iron, diamond, platinum, coal, tin, crude oil, fertile forest etc. including good weather condition yet their governments and presidents spend much of their time going about borrowing and begging from nations who do not have fraction of those natural resources and labor force. They never seem to work toward developing their land mass resources into valuables that will turn their nations around and better the lots of people therein.

Esau - the busy man of the field (hunter) is hungry; Jacob the mild man is cooking stew. Strangely, such is life. It is not all about who is working the more or who is doing the most lucrative job but it is all about that resources that can constantly feed you in the now and in the future. Those resources that will not make you go hungry.

Life is a competition, in other words human beings are competitive in nature. For you to make progress in life, you must plan for the future always. Progress is just like walking, where you take feet ahead of the other continuously until you reach your destination while failure is like trying to take your two feet the same time in the same place. **In the venture of life, your future is either fulfilled or destroyed by the choices you take today and it will have a long way to go with your success line or story.**

The **HUNGRY HUNTER** is an adjective used to qualify the set of hardworking class people or nation blessed with natural resources but have little to show for it or still go about begging for financial assistance either by borrowing or by seeking assistance. Esau's and Jacob's life was used as a case study.

What job are you doing? Are you okay with it? Can it satisfy you for the now and future? Will it feed you when you are hungry?

There are many factors causing hunger as a working class. The factors will be discussed on the subsequent chapters.

CHAPTER 2

FAILURE TO LISTEN TO GOD'S VOICE (Deuteronomy 28:15-23)

One of the factors why you go hungry inspite your income is "failure to listen to God's voice". Let take a look on DEUT. 28:15- 23

15But if you will not obey the voice of the lord your God, being watchful to do all his commandments and his statutes which I command you this day, then all these curses shall come upon you and overtake you

16Cursed shall you be in the city and cursed shall you be in the field.

17Cursed shall be your basket and your kneading trough.

18Cursed shall be the fruit of your body, of your land, of the increase of your cattle and the young of your sheep.

19Cursed shall you be when you come in and cursed shall you be when you go out.

20The lord shall send you curses, confusion, and rebuke in every enterprise you set your hand, until you are destroyed, perishing quickly because of the evil of your doings by which you have forsaken me.

21The lord will make the pestilence cling to you until he has consumed you from the land into which you go to possess.

22The lord will smite you with consumption, with fever and inflammation, fiery heat, sword and drought, blasting and mildew; they shall pursue you until you perish.

[23]The heavens over your head shall be brass and the earth under you shall be iron.

When you fail to listen to God's voice and obey what He commands, there is no amount of work you do in life that will satisfy you for the now and for the future. Rather, your experience will be starvation and your future will be sold out. Esau did not listen to God's voice and that is why the bible referred to him as a profane man Heb. 12:16.

The good news is that God will never consult your past to decide your future. What matters is the renewal of the mindset and by listening to God's voice to observe and to do all is commandments, and then will your field and all you lay hands on will be successful. What guarantees the outpouring of your rain of blessing and sustains you for the now and future, is your absolute obedience to God's voice and instruction. Your miracle, blessing, fulfillment is in that voice and instruction (Gen.28:3, 5-6, 12-13).

Chapter 3

HUNTING WITHOUT ROASTING (prov.12:27)

Esau came from a hunting trip, he probably has meat, and he smells the big pot of stew Jacob has fixed simmering over an open fire. He says "hey Jacob, how about fixing me a bowl of your pottage", Jacob says, "can I tell you what I'll do, I'll trade you a bowl of my stew for your birthright". Esau did not say "No way" or "you have got to be kidding me" or "better still you must be out of your mind". No. Rather he said, "I am about to starve to death what good is my birthright if I am dead" he exaggerated his hunger. Esau could have taken his time to roast his game and process it to eat but he was lazy. One of the reasons why people go hungry, workers go hungry, nations go hungry is because they fail to roast that they took in hunting. Prov. 12:27

27 A lazy man does not roast his game but the diligent man prizes his possession (NIV)

There are many people who are good at hunting, but do not roast what they hunted for. Roasting is the process that takes hunted meat from its raw state into edible state.

- **Hunting** in this context is that job you are doing, it can be professional or not. Like singing, teaching selling etc.
- **Prey or game** is that income, salaries, gain you have in the cause of that job while
- **Roasting** simply means the processing of that you've got from hunting(job) that is (your game or prey) to a secondary product that can add more value and increase than when in a raw state.

Hunting without roasting describes the disposition of those who do not learn to process their primary product into useful secondary product, the resource of a person acquired that does not go through processing; the bible termed such person Lazy. The laziness in this contest does not literally mean idleness (siting doing and doing nothing) but mental laziness, creative laziness, reproductive laziness. The three are from the mind and I call them the Tri-laziness because they are determinant factor for hunger. I guess to you, people who sit around in life and never engage in any demanding activity. That is usually the picture of a 'lazy man' known to you right? Thus, when we see people who are involved in an activity we tend to call them 'hard working' and not lazy. To us, a 'hard working' man or woman, boy or girl cannot be a 'lazy man' at the same time. Yet the verse in the book of proverbs, describes a hunter as a 'lazy man. That disqualify our view of a 'lazy man' and it also entails that there is another characteristics for a 'lazy man's. Let quickly explain the tri-laziness as the characters.

Mental laziness: mental laziness is when someone finds it too tasking to contemplate and explore the possibilities available to him that is beyond his routine.

Creative laziness: Creative laziness is when someone finds it too tasking to make use of is income, salaries or resource (primary product) for a new stream of income flows that will benefit the environment and himself.

Reproductive laziness: Reproductive laziness is when someone finds it too tasking to make use of his primary product to increase and better his lots.

The human mind is a determinant factor for success or failure because mindset represents the choice we make and the choice we make leads to a specific destination of either of the two. A mind that is idle and never get rid of the tri-laziness is a lazy person. We sometimes call them decent hard-working people. They are happy doing one particular thing over and over again and never set their mind into innovation and into new fields. Most hard-working engineers, teachers, doctors, plumbers, and so on, live from day to day, weekends to weekends, month to month, on one particular salary. Anytime salary comes in, it goes out into expenditure. They have never thought of how to make that money to bring forth more money. **A mind preoccupied with laziness can never understand the language of roasting.** The above kinds of laziness are very difficult to detect because most of the people who practice it are very "hardworking" in the contest of real life.

Esau ran with his feet after animal in wild; Jacob with his brain to discover a new and better way to roast (cross breeding) the stock of animals he had to produce a better offspring. **"Those who don't roast that which they took in hunting remain at the level of rawness "by Mensal Otabil"**. Esau had meat with him, he had what it takes not to go hungry, he had what it takes to feed his stomach at the present and to ensure that his future was not tempered with but decided to go for a secondary processed vegetable and meat sauce (pottage). Individual also suffers this same fate as of Esau. The individual who is simply pleased because he has the capacity to produce but does not look at the possibilities of reproduction or processing in what he is doing, will also be running personal deficit like that of Esau. Any individual who sees his or her salary as spending money alone will always run a personal deficit in his/her finance.

There are young people with great talents who allow their present frustration to define their future thereby allowing themselves to be used by their boss_or sponsored and in these causes, they never see themselves as being productive or useful. Their talent just shines through, but their low mentality obscures the shine on their talent. The talent is there but it has not been roasted. Those who roast their value are those who are able to use the power of their mind to design what should happen after today and those who are able to use the power of forward-looking imagination to design how the future will look like. I have a friend who actually put me into track, he told me that his monthly salary is ₦30000 (thirty thousand naira) and what he normally does is, he divides the salary into three parts after removing his tithe and tags them as transportation, feeding and savings respectively. He does this not only to his salary alone but to any money that comes to his hand that is tangible. Within two year, he was able to buy himself a second-hand car which he puts on the road for taxi on daily returns of ₦3000 (three thousand naira). He started with one car but today he has not less than 30(thirty) cars on the road that are giving returns on a daily basis. That is roasting am talking about. After hearing him out, a voice in me told me that my feet are ordered. This friend of mine can never go hungry if his basic salary stops. I also have a brother in the church I attend; I was his best man during his wedding. When I went to board car going to his place during the time of his wedding, I heard people in the park discussing about him. Even all through the journey as we were heading towards his community, he was the subject of discussion. What are they discussing about him? You may be curious to know. They call him small boy that has cars on the road, according to one of them "some of the cars running through Choba Park (that is in Port Harcourt, River State, Nigeria) are owned by him and he is just a plumber". I barely know him very well then and people inside never knew I was going to best this same person they were discussing about. A roaster is known by the numbers of life he/she has affected positively. They don't need to announce themselves because their hand works are evident. What life have you affected positively with your present position?

Do not sell off your future because of an irresponsible appetite; you are absolutely responsible for the outcome of your future. Some leave the place where they sell or utilize their raw product without roasting it and actually thinks they have had pleasure and a good time just like Esau. You can't eat your cake and still have it. People always say "I don't have time, I am an oil worker, what time do I have to set up my own business, this environment I am is too local for the type of business I want to do etc. But the truth is, there is no dry land anywhere, there are only dry mind. That is to say there is no place you cannot process your primary product. It takes a mind full of ideas; creative and productive mindset to look at your environment and know what roasting of your product can mean and what benefits this can bring to you and your environment. Stop saying my environment is not a business area or my environment has nothing to offer me because it is too local. After my encounter with this friend of mine, I now drafted my theory to success "you don't save to spend; you save to invest, you don't save to pleasure; you save to plan" but your profit from the investment should give you the pleasure or spending you need. Many people sold away the value of what would have made them great just for the present pleasure as Esau did.

Another friend of mine who runs his mother's business(school), once told me" Mr. Fidelix, until you discover among all your values the one to put in use, you will never be settled and fulfilled. In other words, his advice to me is to focus on the field that gives me joy and where I am a real specialist. There are people who had talents and never know which of these talents “to roast". Until you discover that which gives you joy and applicable to your environment, you will roast and there will be no visible outcome or you will roast and burn your value.

If you fail to roast that which you took in hunting, poverty is sure to strike at your door because a hungry man is an angry man and an angry man is a poor man. There is no poverty anywhere, it is the laziness of the mind and laziness of the hand that causes poverty (prov.10:4). For you not to be poor and thereby going hungry, you need to put your mind and hand to work. If you fail to roast that game in your possession, a diligent man will negotiate with you leaving you no option but to sell it to him **(prov. 12:27b)** ***“but a diligent man prizes his possession" (NIV).*** **To avoid the mistake Esau did, you need to always put in mind the importance of roasting.**

ADVANTAGES OF ROASTING THAT WHICH YOU GOT FROM HUNTING

- Roasting add value to your product.
- Roasting makes it possible for the usefulness of a product to be preserved for a long time.
- It provides more money than when it is in is raw form.
- It serves as another stream of income.
- It has a taste of time and withstands the test of time.
- Roasting makes you dignified in the community and in what you eat.

To a hungry man who refuses to roast his game, every bitter thing is sweet but the man who roasted that which he took from hunting even honey will be selected. He will always go for the best while the rest will be stepped on. Roasting makes you dignified in the community and in what you eat. Prov. 27:7

"He who is full loathes honey, but to the hungry even what is bitter* taste sweet" *(NIV)

From the above scripture you will see that a hungry man has no option, every option is good because he is hungry but to him that is not hungry takes time to select the best of the best. Esau, because he was hungry and lazy to roast his game, accepts the terms of Jacob which naturally in his right state of mind he will never. Esau people or nations are selling off their rainforest as timber, mineral resources for a pittance just to survive from their present economic hardship. As a Nigerian, it griefs my heart when I see how our crude oil is been exported to be processed only to buy it back at a high price. Can't we get the infrastructure needed for the refining of this crude oil and refine them ourselves? If we don't redesign the structure of our productivity at which we are operating with, Nigeria will continue to experience setbacks. A nation will be poor, if it does not have the capacity to manage its resources from the raw primary product stage to compound stage. Today our young men, women, boys and girls who probably their ideas would have set this great country to a higher standard, are leaving the country for greener pastures, to contribute and build other civilized countries. The economic mishaps in our country today is as a result of not roasting our God given mineral resources in the right way and until we set our priority right, we will continue to go hungry. A country that is hungry, anything brought therein or any negotiation from other country will be accepted because a hungry man has no option. Talking about roasting of your game(value/income), it is not for people/nation with blur vision or immature minds; it is for those mature enough to take risk, advice and see every moment as moment of production of new things.

Our great nation needs to look from this perspective "roasting our mineral resources from primary level (raw form) to secondary level (finishing form) by ourselves" and see if this great country will not turn around for good. A corporate organization, nation or individual who fail to process its value into valuable product can be likened to the lazy hunter who does not process his prey beyond its raw state. Roasting takes place when we take what we have in the raw state through a process that transforms it from a single raw item into a branded and useful item.

Roasting cannot be achieved without heat. The heat for roasting can be likened to the pressure for new training and skill development you put yourself through in order to increase your value. Roasting requires your constant turning of meat so as to prevent a side from burning while the other side remaining raw. This simply means that in processing our values, constant changes and repositioning is needed to make us always fit for the market. What you know today may not be enough for what you want to do tomorrow. Burnt and raw meat are not fit for consumption likewise raw and over exposed talents and products have little market value.

Chapter 4

FAITHFULNESS IN INCREASING OUR VALUE (Matt. 25:26-30)

Faithfulness is not just the ability to preserve that which you have but your ability to increase that which you have. Investing what you have to beget an income is better than keeping it the state you receive it. Life is a test, life is an assignment, life is a business and life is a trust. Some people are simply working hard to keep things as they are and think they are being faithful to God. They insult and mock those ones who try to increase the little value God gave to them and they termed them as being materialistic but they will receive the shock of their life when the Lord will say to them, 'you wicked and lazy servant ... you could have put my talent or value I gave you in the bank and earned some profit on it. (Mat. 25:26-27).

Take a look at the story of my friend I gave previously, his basic salary is N30000 in a month but he invested N9000 for saving every month. In two years, he realizes ₦216000 outside other money he got which was not known to me. He was able to buy a second-hand car which gives him ₦3000 every day. Let's do the mathematics together, in a week of six days he realizes N18000, in a month he realizes N72000. Let just say for maintenance and other expenses he spent ₦12000 then he is left with ₦60000. That is times two of his basic salary in a month. If your income is equal to your expenses then you will be in one position without increase. God wants us to increase in the value He has given to us.

We termed people too materialistic when such people by usury and unjust increased that which they took (game or prey) in hunting. Prov. 28:8, Eccl. 2:26

provide 28:8*He who increases his wealth by exorbitant interest amasses it for another who will be kind to the poor.*

Eccl 2:26*To the man who pleases him, God gives wisdom, knowledge, and happiness but the sinner he gives the tasks of gathering and storing up wealth to hand over to the one who pleases God. This is too meaningless, a chasing after the wind.*

From the scriptures above, people who increase his value by just means, God gives wisdom, understanding in their roasting and also rest of mind (happiness) but to the unjust, such people end up serving people instead of people serving them. They even end up losing that which they gather through struggling. Such people will gather but their gathering is like the wind.

In the scripture, Matt. 25:26-30, you will see that life is a business (my second book yet to be published; **LIFE AS A BUSINESS**), that is why when Esau and Jacob meet at the negotiation table, the outcome are different for the both of them. It was a trade by barter business. One uses the value he has to buy the value he desires of (birthright) while the other uses the value he despised to buy d present need so as to feed himself. What are you negotiating for and what are you buying? (Prov. 23:1), Does it increase your value for the future or it satisfies thy need for the moment alone.

Generation of Jacob applies God's law of increase. God's law simply means set of rules and standard issued by God.

Lev. 26:3-5. ***If ye work in my statues and keep my commandments and do them.***

I will give you rain in due season, and the land shall yield her increase and the trees of the field their fruit.

And your threshing time shall reach to the vintage and the vintage time shall reach the sowing time, and you shall eat you bread to the full and dwell in your land securely*.*

Jacob understands these principles and his substance increases. **You know when God seems you don't deserve a particular thing; you can actually quote his law to move his hand.**

God's law of increase simply means a set of rules and standard issued by God to make you expand or increase in all you do in life. God's law of increase works with the law of giving *(Prov. 11:24-25). This* portion of the bible says,***"there is that scatereth, yet increaseth, and there is that withholdeth more than is met, but it tendereth to poverty. The liberally soul shall be made fat; and he that watereth shall be watered also himself".*** Jacob knowing this principle of giving (scattering) that is why he gave out his pottage knowing very well that the pottage will surely be harvested in multiple fold in the long run while Esau, having prey at hand but fail to roast it thereby withholding it and this cost him a fortune. When you fail to apply God's law of increase, you are toeing the path of poverty and you will go hungry. If you hold on to money or value tight without investment, you will lose it. God's law of increase does not always make sense. The measure of your faith toward giving determines the increase of your harvest (Luke 6:38) **"give and it shall be given unto you; good measure, pressed down, and shaken together, and running over, shall men give into your bosom. For the same measure that ye mete withal it shall be measured to you again".** The biblical illustration talks more on the deal of Esau. And Jacob gave pottage to Esau; Jacob received his blessing after the pottage he gave to his father has been eaten by the father Isaac **(Gen. 27:1-5).**

"And Esau went to the field to hunt for venison and to bring it to his father. Gen. 27:5b" *D*efinitely he will roast and garnish it forgetting that he has traded this roasting for these blessing long ago. The measure in which you take life, will surely be the same measure that will return back to you. If you see what you have as useless when the time for the value to be useful comes, you will loss it (you will not have access to it). Expectation is the mother of manifestation. As a man thinketh in his heart so is he. Chances can be taken because God is purpose and time oriented. Jacob gave pottage to Esau to buy his birthright, Jacob uses that same pottage (which is now a document) to receive blessing from his father. Every negotiation towards increase is a give and take affair (barter). You offer what you have for what you need. Anyone who negotiates with Jacob's generation must be careful of what they ask for. If Esau had known that his negotiation will lead to losing his birthright, he won't have agreed to the terms and condition rather he will take time to roast his value (game). Be careful of your negotiation for the satisfactory of now.

Hunger is not good for children of God because if you are hungry, you can't serve God effectively. Poverty and hunger are brothers and sister because a poor man is a hungry man. You can be rich and be hungry then you are poor. **Until you take dominion over poverty and laziness of the mind, hunger is a sure thing**. As a child of God, you need not to be poor because God's lineage (blood) is flowing in us and since is flowing in us, we need to take charge of increase in our value (2Corinth. 8:9) ***"for ye know the grace of the lord Jesus Christ, that***

though he was rich, yet for your sakes he became poor, that ye through is poverty might be rich". Money and riches are relative term. Money is the resource (value), God is the source. Obedience and faithfulness to the source guarantee the flow of the resources to increase. The following factors guarantee dominion (increase) over poverty.

FAITHFULNESS IN TITHE: Tithe is giving God what belongs to him. It can also be said to be one tenth of your income (Malachi 3:10). Your faithfulness in tithing makes your value to increase and also makes you to be satisfy and not go hungry but when you are not faithful in tithe, then you are cursed by God (Malachi. 3:8-9). Nothing you do in the field that will prosper. This simply means you will struggle like an Elephant, eat like an Ant.

If you must increase in your value then you must take dominion over poverty and also practicing the law of increase. Don't forget God's law of increase "**whatever a man sows, that he will reap**". When you make wrong choices in life, you receive the consequences of the choices in time to come; it might be short or long. Increase that which you have and see God giving you more. **An uncommon seed always creates an uncommon harvest**. When you receive your salary or income, ask yourself these questions:

- What do I have?
- What do I do with what I have?
- Will I consume or invest it?
- What do I invest it on?
- Can I get more from what I have than what I am now getting?
- Do I have the information and skills to increase my investment?

- Can I be patient enough to see my investment turn into a valuable yield?

Your honest answer to this question will help you discover the potential and possible achievement in what is in your hand. The key to increase earning capacity is to develop very valuable skills. A man's income in life is contingent on the amount of good he can do to his generation and the quantitative and qualitative contribution to humanity (Jim Rohn).

He was poor so that we can be rich, increase and multiply. Increase is a need for people or nation whose bloodline is that of Jesus Christ.

Chapter 5

FEAR

(Deal with It before It Disvalues Your Value)

Fear is the dark room where people develop their negative potentials. Many people live in constant fear, they are scared of whom they are, of what they want to become and they are scared of failure and whosoever is scared of failure, will never attain success. Fear is the constant feeling of depressed emotion. When you allow fear to eat much into you, you will be stagnant in one place, you might even sell your future there because you will be afraid of moving forward and even scared of taking a step backward thereby ready at that point to take the available plane to relief you of your fear; resulting on a negotiation. Human beings set a limitation or imaginary boundaries for themselves because of fear of exploiting. If you don't launch your goal because of fear, nobody will do it for you remember that nobody congratulates a pregnant woman, but people will always celebrate her when she put to bed regardless of the pain she passes through. If you don't conquer your fear, it will dominate you and turn you to a slave of your talent. Remember Apostle Paul's letter to Timothy it says ***"for God has not given us a spirit of fear, but of power and love and of a sound mind***".

Life here on earth is full of uncertainty, thereby imposing fear on humans on how to survive including Christians. Esau, having meat at hand, was afraid that before he roasts and garnish it into edible form, he will die but if he had thrown away fear or not being anxious of him dying, probably the negotiation won't have taken place. Worry, anxiety, fear are all synonymous in meaning.

According to one of my fathers in the lord Rev. Nwonzuzu, he defines worry as over speeding of a car or overloading of a car. If you overload your mind or heart with worries, you will sink or breakdown just as a car will when overloaded. When you are so worry about the future without any plan of roasting that you have for the future, you will wear out or loose brake just like Esau. Esau broke down when he discovered his birthright has been taken by his brother Jacob as a result of their negotiation in the past. Fear is a cripple disease that eats gradually into you and lodges you into darkness; don't overload, over speed or exaggerate your life like Esau did. Fear is a depressor to your achievement, if being considered; it can either slow you down or stop you. Overcoming your worries will liberate you to achieving your destiny. Never let your mind settle for the spirit of fear because it will reduce you to naught. This story illustrates it better

"A mouse was in constant distress because of its fear of Cat. A magician took pity on it and turn it into a cat but then it became afraid of the Dog: The magician turned it into a dog, then he began to be afraid of the Panther, the magician also turned it into a panther, where upon it was full of fear for the hunter" at this point the magician gave up and turned it back into a mouse saying "nothing I do for you is going to be of any help because you have the heart of a mouse". God has given many of you three different talents on three different occasion but you fail to put it into roasting to yield productivity all because of fear and thereby making God to give up on you. God will never give up on you in Jesus name (Amen). My reader, you have to deal with your fear. Are you battling with some of your problems because you are scared? They will always be there and you can't do without them? Is your struggling to be great in life but right inside your mind you are afraid of making step so you settle yourself for the level of mediocre? You might look like a lion, you might change your appearance but if you don't change your mind from that of a mouse to that of a lion, you will forever be lost in the battle of "fear of failure" which will hinder you from succeeding. How can you be great if your mind doesn't portrait what you are fighting for? I was once filled with fear of the uncertainty but I started to change by changing my mind to that of a lion, taming my fear and changing my perspective.

Relating with our core scripture and characters, Esau was thinking he will die if he doesn't eat at that time (he was unable to control himself) but we all know that that is a fallacy. If he had dealt with his fear, he wouldn't have negotiated his future for a mere pottage. Likewise, our nation Nigeria, needs right perspectives to actually see that all her economic (values) she has, are being used to build up a standard refinery (roasting). Though it will shake us but the end result will be wow. When the going gets tough, tough men keep going and that is what makes them great. Do you want to be great? Keep moving in that your challenge. If there is anybody to be feared, it should be GOD. Psalm 112:1-3 "***praise ye the lord. Blessed is the man that feareth the lord that delights greatly in His commandment. His seed shall be mighty upon the earth; the generation of the upright shall be blessed. Wealth and riches shall be in his house and his righteousness endureth forever***". Even when your life seems to be leaving you, don't give room for fear in other not to disvalue your value (ps. 23:4). Put your anchor on Christ because in your week point, he will substitute His strength for your weakness. Hear me my reader no problem that cometh your way arrives before the solution. God makes us great because we are no more but in him so why the fear? A Christian who cannot do away with fear cannot evaluate his/her life and a Christian who cannot evaluate his/her life is bound to fail. Whenever there is consternation, just kneel down to God and pray. Kneels of a solid

Christian is powerful than the concoction made by the evil and wicked people of the day. Be conscientious to do away with fear when it comes knocking. All trouble, situation and problem you face are common so why the fear? For you to overcome fear, you must have courage.

Courage requires that you make yourself do what you should do, that you deal with your fears rather than avoiding them.

The biggest obstacle to success in life is fear of failure, expressed in the feeling that, "I can't! I can't! I can't!" but summon courage.

Courage is a habit, developed by practicing courage whenever it is required.

As Emerson said, "Do the thing you fear and the death of fear is certain."

Make a habit of confronting your fears rather than avoiding them. When you confront the fear and move toward it, especially if it is another person or people or situation, the fear gets smaller and you become braver.

Repeat the words to cancel fear, "I can do it!" over and over, to build up your courage and confidence.

Identify one fear in your life and then within yourself deal with it as you confront it doing whatever it involves, as quickly as you possibly can. The payoff for identifying a fear and confronting it is tremendous, it gives you the courage and confidence to go through your life and deal with every fear-inducing situation.

The fear of the Lord is the beginning of wisdom: a good understanding has all they that do his commandments: his praise endured forever. Psalm 111:10

The fear of the Lord is a basic requirement for any Christian wishing to triumph in life. It is also of vital importance to anyone who desires to register in the school of wisdom. The man, who walks in the fear of the Lord, has automatic access to supernatural wisdom. This is where to begin from in your quest for wisdom.

Look at Joseph in chapter 41 of Genesis, wisdom lifted him to a position of authority, and he became a ruler in the land of Egypt.
And Pharaoh said unto Joseph, Forasmuch as God hath shewed thee all this, there is none so discreet and wise as thou art: Thou shalt be over my house, and according unto thy word shall all my people be ruled: only in the throne will I be greater than thou.
And Pharaoh said unto Joseph, See, I have set thee over all the land of Egypt. Genesis 41:39-41.

But he enrolled in the school of wisdom by possessing the fear of the Lord. He said, " ... how then can I do this great wickedness, and sin against God?" (Genesis 39:9.) And also, "... For I fear God"(Genesis 42:18).

Daniel also arrived on the scene and would not defile himself with the king's rich food; therefore, God lifted him. Any man can be distinguished and enthroned on the earth today, if he will part ways with sin. Loyalty to serving God without committing sin is what gives you access to the instructions of wisdom which lead to your celebration on earth.

What man is he that feared the LORD? him shall he teach in the way that he shall choose.

The secret of the LORD is with them that fear him; and he will show them his covenant. Psalm 25:12,14.
Finally know that: fear need to be conquered in the following ways:

- By prayer and supplication (phil. 4:6)
- Committing your way and your business or work to his hand
- Above all faith. Esau never has faith that is why he gave way for fear.

My reader, tame your fear, change your mind, change your perspective and rule your world.

Chapter 6

LACK OF INFORMATION

The search for opportunities is infinity. These opportunities are utilized variously through different means. One of such means is **information**. Information is a processed data. It makes sense and it serves as awareness. According to Ola Oluwa "an expedition to the world of insight or imagination becomes inevitable." There is a poem considered very meaningful and relevant for the purpose of these heading. It is titled "Diamond in the Rough".

A diamond in the rough
Is a diamond sure enough
For before it ever sparkled
It was made diamond stuff
Of course someone must find it
Or it never will be found
And then, someone must grind it
Or it never will be grinded
When it burnishes bright
That diamond will be everlasting
Flashing out its radiant light.

Just as diamond exist in the rough, so does treasure exist in information. As the rough is processed in other to bring out of it the diamond, so should information be processed to bring out the treasure there in. When information is adapted as useful working tool or success working tools, thinking capability sharpens, vocabulary will improve and success working life will become more interesting. The new source of power is not money in the hand of few but information in the hand of many. If Esau had sought information on the proposal of his brother (Jacob) from his father (Isaac), probably he won't have sold his birthright but because he lacked information on the proposal from

Jacob, he sold his birthright not knowing the consequences. You can predict your future by the awareness you have of your purpose. **Too many people know what they are running from but not where they are running to**. Esau runs away from preparing himself pottage from his game because he was hungry and he try to avoid the hunger stuff and never knew his action would lead him to selling his future. According to Jim Rohn, "Up until the age of twenty-five, I worked hard on my job and I made a living. Starting at the age of twenty-five, I worked hard on myself and I made a fortune" thus his lesson is "success is not something you pursue. Success is something you attract because of the person you become". If only Esau had worked hard on himself, he won't have faced that big loses. You see what we need to a successful life is information. Thomas Carlyle states that **I**ngenuity requires **I**nformation, **I**nformation determines the depth of the **I**dea that runs through the proportion of **I**ncome to be attracted by an individual

INGENUITY INFORMATION IDEA INNOVATION INCOME

You will notice that in between **I**'s word lies **IDEA** and it is the idea that we need in all our doing and to make a difference. If only Esau have this idea (roasting that which he took from hunting), his birthright would have not been negotiated for a pottage. *When information is adopted as a tool for work, it would be discovered that there is more of:* ***Brain work thinking*** *and less of* ***field work activity****. Thinking is very essential because whatever the mind can conceive and believe will eventually be achieved.* John Mason remarks "think only for the best, work only for the best and expect only the best". Excellence is never an accident. If Esau had thought of processing his game to pottage, he would have had enough to eat, give to his father, mother and probably Jacob too and his mind won't have gone that shallow to accepting selling his birthright. The four lepers in the bible took information down to the children of Israel and the children of Israel never neglected the information irrespective of the people that brought it down to them. The outcome settles famine at that time. Use the information you have heard, read and you will see, you will never be hungry again.

In today's economy, the race that makes us strong is the race at which we process the information available before us and how we use the information to accomplish tasks assigned to us. "It is not so much you know but how quickly you translate what you know into what you do" (Mensa otabil). There is a saying that readers are potential leaders. This is absolutely correct, looking at it from a different perspective Ola-Oluwa states in his book "although readers are potential leaders, it is often time when this statement is made, it relates to leader in terms of positional or hierarchical capacity. As much as this is important or true, equally important is the fact that it should be from the perspective that leaders are those who BLAZE THE TRIAL in their chosen job, carrier or field". These are those who take risks or operate on the fringe of life. Thus trail-blazing is a pre-requisite for leadership. This is what really makes reader potential leader. When you get information, filter the idea therein by getting expertise before embarking on roasting of your game. You don't have to do it yourself what you need is to invest in expert who can deliver. When it was time for Isaac to bless his first-born Esau, he called him to the living room and instructed him on what to do but Rebecca heard it and gave the information to Jacob but Jacob doesn't know how to make venison for Isaac his father such as is soul love. Rebecca went further to tell Jacob don't worry I will take charge of everything. Sometime when information gets to us we don't need to do it ourselves. People or nation who uses Jacob system, don't try to do it themselves when they can receive experts' help. Jacob teamed up with his mother (practicing expert), who was an expert in preparing for Isaac meals "such as my soul loves" and Isaac on the other hand don't know the difference between home breed meat and bush meat because expert is at work. Expert who knows what to do, don't beat about the bush when serious information is at hand with experimentation at your expense.

DO YOU WANT FISH OR HOW TO CATCH FISH

Lazy people don't need information to greatness rather they need instant breakthrough. Some people don't want to know how to avoid hunger but they need food to avert their hunger. If you read the bible verse with close view, you will notice that Esau's request is an instructive one. He says to Jacob; '***give me some of the same stew you are eating'***. He wanted the same 'roasted' resources of Jacob in its processed form. He was not looking for information on how to cook his own food e.g he was not looking for fire, recipe of Jacob stew, and ingredients rather he just wants the finish product of Jacob and not the means to process his raw game into edible food. People like Esau are people or nations who are lazy and desperate to eat fish without learning or knowing how to catch one. They have no time and discipline to get the recipe for what they desire and cook it themselves. Esau kind of person or nations like to partake on people's success without considering its possible cost. What Esau people fail to understand is that those who uses their time and skill to put a raw material into finished products have high price for their goods and services. They don't sell it cheap.

When you don't make use of information at your hand and you are expecting someone else processed information for instant gratification, you will have little patience for wisdom, tact and good judgement. Infact your hunger becomes a trap for you. Any good negotiator will tell you that overzealous and eager traders easily loss out in negotiation. Don't wait for people to feed you rather look for information on what will feed you. As a worker you don't eat until you are paid, you can't even cook your desire meal because you are cutting down your needs due to insufficiency. Process your information and stop depending on already processed information.

Chapter 7

FAILURE TO LIVE A LIFE OF FULFILMENT

The desire to get ahead makes all of us competitive. As human beings, we challenge ourselves to see what we are capable of doing and challenge others to find out whether we can do better than them.

To become someone in life, you must face challenges and the challenges are examination to your success of next level. Your response to those challenges determines your success or failure. This world is an examination center. The fact is, no one escapes from it; thus, to become great or successful, you must sit down to pass your exams. When I look at life of fulfillment generally, people desire to have good and successful life of fulfillment without the readiness to pass exams of challenges. What this means is that:

- One who is expecting to build a house without proper planning.
- One who is expecting to harvest healthy crop that your generation will benefit from after without proper cultivation, and proper care of the seed sown.
- One attempting to use electrical devices without power supply.

Examination is defined as a test of a student's knowledge or skills in a particular subject or matter which results in a qualification. The battle of success is not won by struggling, they are won by strategies. The more you look at your background maybe at your family background, present situation, the more you are prevented from moving. Your family background cannot stop you or cannot be a challenge to you but the You in You can stop you and make the background a realistic evidence in your life. You can only be satisfied with your life if you live it in Christ Jesus otherwise crises will make it miserable. If you have to satisfy your hunger in any way, do not let your hunger to show. Tame it, in fact be discipline when you are hungry, be discipline about your need and be discipline about your present need to avoid living a miserable life. In life, there is always a purpose for everything that exists in our world. Dr Myles Munroe of blessed memory once said that when the purpose of a thing is not known, abuse is inevitable. Esau failed his life examination to a fulfilled life because he lacked self-confidence which I will discuss on later, and he is of course a profane man even though he begged to resist for that examination with tears. He never knew the importance of life examination. Heb. 12:16-17

That no one should become guilty of sexual vice, or become a profane (godless and sacrilegious) person as Esau did, who sold his own birthright for a single meal.

For you understand that later on, when he wanted (to regain title to) his inheritance of blessing, he was rejected (disqualified and set aside), for he could find no opportunity for repair by repentance (what he has done, no chance to recall the choice he had made), although he sought for it carefully with (bitter) tears. (AMP)

Esau lived a life outside God and his life was miserable. Living a life of fulfillment needs a life that is hungry for God and not a life that is hungry and conscious of the present need for self-aggrandizement. Esau's life is likened to be the generation who fought for a fulfilled life by struggling while that of Jacob is likened to strategy. It takes a life who knows God to have strategy that will make him work less before success is achieved. Burial ground ever remains the richest place in the world. Why? Because there, lays so much virgin potentials, kings that never reigned, pastors that never fulfilled their ministry, presidents that never presided, Doctors that never attended to any patient, professors that never professed until they died. All because they never put their priority right, they lived a wasted life. You can be a Christian and still live a wasted life that is if you don't put your priority right by putting in use your potentials to solve environment, community, country and world needs. Don't be a wasted life like Esau who never set his priority right. Every human being was created for a specific purpose in life and such a person is embedded with value to actualize that purpose. No one is born without a reason and no one comes to the world for coming sake. Moses was born when God saw that there was a need for Moses to be used for the deliverance of Israel. Samson too was born when there was need for someone to deliver Israel from the hand of the philistines. God has plan for every hand he has put in place and it can only be made manifest if only we know our value and tame our hunger for the present.

Many people measure fulfillment in terms of worldly achievements; what a big mistake. Esau later on was liberated and he was rich but he was never fulfilled because his birthright was never regained and that always make his heart bitter. **Fulfillment is measured using God's value in your life in relation to solving economic problems (roasting).** There is a purpose for every individual in life to fulfill. Every item manufactured is designed for a specific purpose and being use otherwise will lead to abuse.

A pen is made for the purpose of writing and the value of the pen is the ink, when you buy one and it does not do the work for which it is made then it is useless because it has not fulfilled what it's made for. All effort in packing and selling it becomes a waste. A man or nation who does not live to fulfill what God has created him for, is just like that ball pen that refuses to write (useless). Everything God has made in life has a purpose of creation and a value to actualize the purpose. He made the sun to shine providing the sun with an inexhaustible helium/oxygen gas, the moon to shine in the night with the help of the sun, and he made human being to have dominion over all creatures of the universe by giving us potentials He (God) possesses. He made us in His own image so we possess his potentials/ power to dominate. When you refuse to do that God created you for, you are resigning being useful.

A pen that refuses to write, a cutlass that refuses to cut all becomes useless. It does not mean it has ceased from existing but it becomes an ordinary thing likewise a man who is living but not fulfilling his ministry (he will be ignored) that is, he becomes valueless and useless. To live a successful life or fulfilled life, you must put in mind the following:

- Success/fulfillment is not by struggling but by strategy (your strategy can only be struggle-free if you know God almighty).
- Discover the purpose for which you are created.
- Don't be a useless material meant for the dustbin nor like that of a ball pen that refuse to write and a cutlass that is blunt and can't cut anything.
- Process the values you have to a finished product.
- Don't sell your value in raw state for the present hunger.

"Your decision in life makes or mars you. When it is wrongly made, you destroy a destiny" (Evang. Ominije J.K). At the journey of living a life of fulfillment, you have a choice to make according to Evang. Ominije J.K "either to obey God fully, or to obey God partially, or better still not to obey God at all but bear in mind that whichever way you choose, have a long way effect to your vision in fulfilling your destiny".

To live a life of fulfillment, stability of mind is very important. When the mind is stable, challenges become a thing to deal with.

Finally **give all your worries and cares to God because He cares for you (1peter. 5:7)**. Dear brothers and sisters, fathers and mothers reading this book; whenever problems/challenges come your way, let it be an opportunity for joy. For when your faith is tested, your endurance has a chance to grow so let it grow for when your endurance is fully developed, you will be strong in character and ready for anything (James. 1:2-4). Living a life of fulfillment will be easy and stress free.

Chapter 8

SELF DISCIPLINE

Self-discipline is different from discipline. Self-discipline is a self-imposed standard; a restriction motivated by a passion that is more than the desire. It is created by power of choice. Until you have taken yourself to that level, you will destroy your destiny.

Proverbs 25:28 ***he that hath no rule over his own spirit is like a city that is broken down, and without walls.***

If you don't want to go hungry, you must develop the habit of self-discipline. Be disciplined even with your money and materials. The best victory to ever achieve is victory to conquer self.

Judas Iscariot conquered everybody but failed in conquering self so money conquered him.

Moses conquered everyone except himself so anger conquered him.

Your ability to develop the habit of self-discipline will contribute more to your success than any other quality of character.

Some years ago, I read a book from a notable and successful author that had discovered one thousand success principles which he had published in four books containing 250 principles each.

Napoleon Hill, after interviewing 500 of the richest people in America, concluded that "Self-discipline is the master key to riches."

Among the thousand principles, he considered self-discipline to be the most.

"The ability to make yourself do what you should do, when you should do it, whether you feel like it or not." when you do things at your own convenient time then you will always settle for averageness or poverty certainly not success.

Al Tomsik said, "Success is tons of discipline."

Dr. Edward Banfield from Harvard concluded that "Long time perspective" was the key to upward social and economic mobility in America or anywhere else in the world.

Esau lacks self-discipline and that is why he could not take time to roast his game, he could not control is appetite for food.

Jim Rollins said, "Discipline weighs ounces, but regret weights tons."

He discovered in fifty years of research, that people who succeeded greatly had the ability to think long term, to delay gratification in the short term so that they could enjoy even greater rewards in the long term. They thought ten and twenty years into the future while making decisions for their current actions. That was Jacob set of people.

"Discipline weighs ounces, but regret weighs tons."

The key word is "sacrifice." It is the ability for you to sacrifice immediate pleasure or gratification in the present so that you can enjoy greater rewards in future.

Esau failed to sacrifice time and that lead to his regret afterward while Jacob sacrifice pottage he has taken his time to make for birthright. What are you sacrificing for the other? Will you regret it or be happy later on? Your action to discipline is proportional to your success later on life.

Albert Einstein once said that: "Compound interest is the most powerful force in the universe."

This is why roasting (saving and investing) in the present is the first key to becoming financially successful in the future.

Self-discipline means self-control, self-mastery, and the ability to have dinner before dessert.

This doesn't mean that you don't have pleasurable experiences in life, but it means that you have them after you have done the hard and necessary work, and completed your key tasks.

The payoff for practicing self-discipline is immediate. Whenever you discipline yourself, and force yourself to do the right thing, whether you feel like it or not, you will like and respect yourself more. Your self-esteem increases. Your self-image improves. Your brain releases

endorphins which made you happy and proud. You actually get a payoff every time you hold your own feet to the fire.
Esau felt birthright does not mean anything and it cannot be compared to his hunger. He cannot hold his hunger thereby allowing his self-image and esteem to decrease.
The most important point is that self-discipline is a habit that you can learn with practice and repetition.
It takes approximately twenty-one days of repetition, without exception, to develop a habit of medium complexity. Sometimes you can develop a habit faster, and sometimes it will take longer. It is up to you, and how determined you are.
Some years ago, a business man, Herbert Grey, began searching for what he called "The common denominator of success."
He researched and interviewed successful people for eleven years and finally concluded that:
Successful people are those who "Make a habit of doing what unsuccessful people don't like to do."
And what are these things? It turns out that successful people don't like to do them either, but they do them anyway, because they realize it is the price of success.
They are people who roast their product even when it's not easy.
There are some types of discipline you can develop that will improve every area of your life. It turns out that every exercise of self-discipline strengthens every other discipline at the same time, just as every weakness in self-discipline weakens you in other disciplines as well and they are.

The Discipline of Clear Thinking/ Decision check:

The essence of decision check / clear thinking cannot be over emphasized. You wouldn't consume anything let say meal except you believed it was prepared in a hygiene environment, would you?
Thomas Edison once said, "Thinking is the hardest discipline of all."

It has been said that there are three types of people. There are those who think (The small minority); there are those that think they think, then there are those who would rather die than think. Take time to think through the critical issues and problems in your life. Put a side long, unbroken chunks of time, thirty, sixty and then ninety minutes. Exercising decision check or clear thinking in your decision making, will have a long-term effect to your life. Do you know that the value you have for your decision over your value will determine your final decision on what to do with it.

Peter Drucker said that, "Fast people decisions are usually wrong people decisions." In addition, fast decisions with regard to your family, career, money or any other major issue are usually wrong decisions.

Sit quietly for 30-60 minutes to think. Practice solitude on a regular basis.

"Go into the silence." Whenever you practice solitude for more than thirty minutes, you activate your super conscious mind and trigger your intuition. You get it right from the "still, small, silent voice within." To think better, take a pad of paper and write down every detail of the problem situation you are facing. Sometimes, the right thing to do immerges as you write down the details.

Aristotle once said that wisdom (The ability to make good decisions) is a combination of experience plus reflection. The more time that you take to think about your experiences, the more vital lessons you will gain from them. Go for a walk or exercise for 30-60 minutes. Very often when you are exercising, you will get insights or ideas that help you to think better and make better decisions.

Talk your situation over with someone else who you like and trust, and who is not emotionally involved. Very often, a different perspective can totally change your viewpoint.

Always ask, "What are my assumptions?" What is it that you are assuming to be true about the situation?

Fast people decisions are usually wrong people decisions. Esau was very fast in answering Jacob and his response actually tie him down on the day he was supposed to received his blessing

What if your assumptions were wrong? What if you were preceded on the basis of false information?

Always be open to the possibility that you could be completely wrong in your current course of action. Be open to doing something completely different.

The discipline of daily Goal-Setting:

Focus and concentration are the essential qualities for success.

Start by asking, "What do I really want to do with my life?" Ask this question over and over again until you get a clear answer. If you don't get clear answer, you will end up earning to balance check your expenses better still go hungry. Imagine that you had ten-million-naira cash, but only ten years to live. What would you immediately do differently in your life? Imagine that you have no limitations. That you could wave a magic wand and have all the time and money, all the education and experience, all the contacts you needed to achieve any goal. What would you do then?

Buy a spiral notebook and write in it every day. Begin by writing out ten goals in the present, positive and personal tense. Begin each goal with the word "I" followed by an action verb.

For example, you could write, "I earn ₦xxxxx.xxx by December 31, 2018."

Every day before you start off, rewrite your top ten goals in the present tense, as though you had already achieved them and you were reporting on this success to someone else. Rewrite your goals without looking back to the previous page.

Rewrite them from memory. Watch how they grow, develop and change over time as you rewrite them each day. Many people have said that the discipline of daily goal setting has transformed their life and far faster than they had even imagined.

The discipline of Daily Time Management:

Rule: "Every minute spent in planning saves ten minutes in execution." The more you plan, the better you use your time, and the more you accomplish.

Begin by making a list of everything that you have to do. The best time to write your daily list is the night before so that your subconscious can work on it while you sleep. Organize the list by priority before starting work. Practice the 80/20 rule, which says that 80% of your results come from 20%of your activities. What are they? Use the ABCDE method to set your time management:

A = Must do – serious consequences for non-completion
B = should do – mild consequences for non-completion
C = Nice to do – no consequences for non-completion
D = Delegate – everything possible
E = Eliminate – everything you can to free up more time

Organize your list by A-1, A-2, A-3, and so on. Start on your A-1 task first thing in the morning.

Discipline yourself to concentrate single-mindedly on your A-1 task until it is 100% complete. The discipline of good time management spreads to all your other disciplines.

The ABCDE time check principle will help you in time management when planning the day, and also realize that there are common time wasters which are:

1. Social media
2. Visitors
3. Irrelevant meeting

4. Paperwork
5. Handset

The Discipline of Saving regularly and Investing:

Emotion should not be allowed to take the place of objective and logical reasoning when it comes to investment. Esau was emotionally not stable because of hunger and he sold out his life investment. Resolve today to get out of debt, stay out of debt and become financially independent. Your goal and everyone's goal is to achieve financial independence as soon as possible in life. This requires continuous financial discipline with every Naira you earn. The key is for you to save 5%, 10% and even 25% of your income throughout your life.

Because you are probably in debt already, begin by saving 1% of your income after you must have paid your tithe and discipline yourself to live on the other 99% until this becomes a habit. Increase the amount of monthly savings to 2%, 3% and eventually 10% and 15%. Discipline yourself to live on the balance. Rewire your thinking from "I enjoy spending" to "I enjoy saving."

Delay; defer major purchases for 30 days. Investigate before you invest. Two thirds of investment success come from avoiding mistakes. Invest as much time in studying the investment as you invested to earn the money in the first place. "If you cannot save money, the seeds of greatness are not in you." (W. Clement Stone)

The Discipline of Continuous Learning: "To earn more you must learn more."

On the road to success, speed limit does not matter. What matters is self-development.

Read relevant book in your field 30-60 pages each day. This will translate into one book per week, 4 book a month.

Attend seminars and take courses given by experts in your field. One idea from one course can save you years of hard work.
The average income of a Nigerian vocational enterprise increases by 3 percent annually. With compound interest, the average person doubles their income every 22 years.
With the additional knowledge and skill you can apply to get better results, you increase your income at 10%, 15% and even 25% per year.
• 10% per annum increase means that you double your income in 7.2 years.
• 25% increase per annum means that you double your income in 2 years and 8 months.
Work on yourself as if your future depends on it, because it does.
Jim Rowan: "Work at least as hard on yourself as you do on your work.

The Discipline of Persistence:
The greatest test of self-discipline is when you persist in the face of adversity, and you drive yourself forward to complete your tasks 100%, no matter how you feel.

Being close to a river bank doesn't nearly translate to drinking and getting refreshed by the water. Making a decision to invest your value does not really means you have make an investment but kick starting it really is investment.

Courage has two parts: The first part is the courage to begin, to start, to launch forward with no guarantees of success. The second part is the courage to endure, to persist, when you feel discouraged and want to quit.
Your persistence is the measure of your belief in yourself, and in what you are doing.
The more you believe in the goodness and rightness of what you are doing, the more you will persist.

The more you persist, the more you will tend to believe in yourself and what you are doing. The principles are reversible! Persistence is actually self-discipline in action.
Self-discipline leads to self-esteem, a greater sense of personal power, which leads to greater persistence, which leads to even greater self-discipline in an upward spiral. "Persistence is to the character of man or woman as carbon is to steel." (Napoleon Hill). You actually make yourself into a better, stronger person by persisting when you feel like quitting. You take complete control over the development of your own character. Eventually, you become unstoppable. "Persistence is actually self-discipline in action."

The benefits of practicing self-discipline in every area of your life are many:

1. The habit of self-discipline virtually guarantees your success in life, both with others and with yourself.
2. You will get more done, faster and of higher quality with discipline than with any other skill.
3. You will be paid more and promoted faster.
4. You will experience a greater sense of self-control, self-reliance and personal power.
5. Self-discipline is the key to self-esteem, self-respect and personal pride.
6. The greater yourself discipline, the greater your self-confidence and the lower will be your fear of failure and rejection. Nothing will stop you.
7. With self-discipline, you will have the strength of character to persist over all obstacles until you eventually succeed.

Begin today to practice self-discipline in every area of your life. Persist in this practice until self-discipline comes to you as automatically and as easily as breathing in and breathing out. Your future will be guaranteed.

ABOUT THE BOOK

If you make smart moves, you can stay away from danger, but any bad decision could be your last. As Christians it is compulsory to identity oneself so as not to go hungry and not regret the action of not knowing/understanding your value. In this book, author Alabi Fidelix explain in details various way you can discover you and your value and ways you can safeguard your future without your present situation disvaluing it.

ABOUT THE AUTHOUR

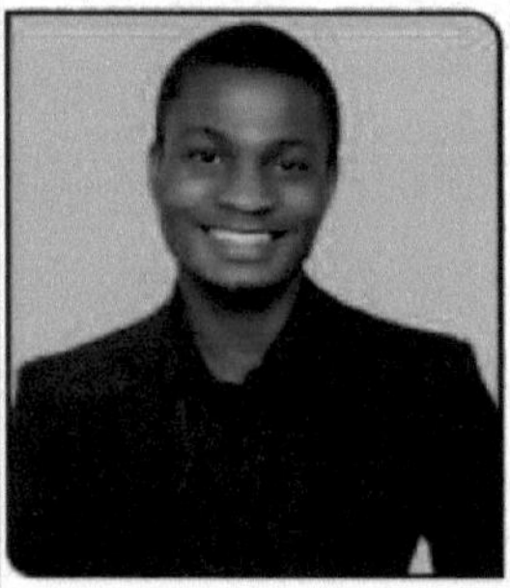

Alabi Fidelix is an Author;
A Motivational Speaker,
A Mathematicians,
A Teacher,
An Engineer (Electrical/Electronics).
Youth President of PS Assembly of Gospel Faith Mission Int'l (GOFAMINT) Port Harcourt.